Green Mental Health Care

How to Get Off & Stay Off Psychiatric Drugs

A Non-Toxic, Non-Invasive, & Non-Addictive Approach

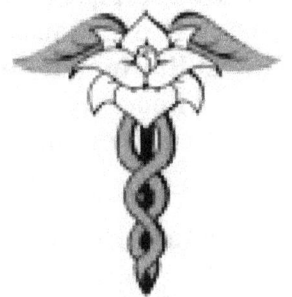

Staying Sane in a Toxic World

Genita M. Mason **H.H.P., N.C., M.H.**
Medical Director, The Biosanctuary
A Green Body & Mind Medical Model

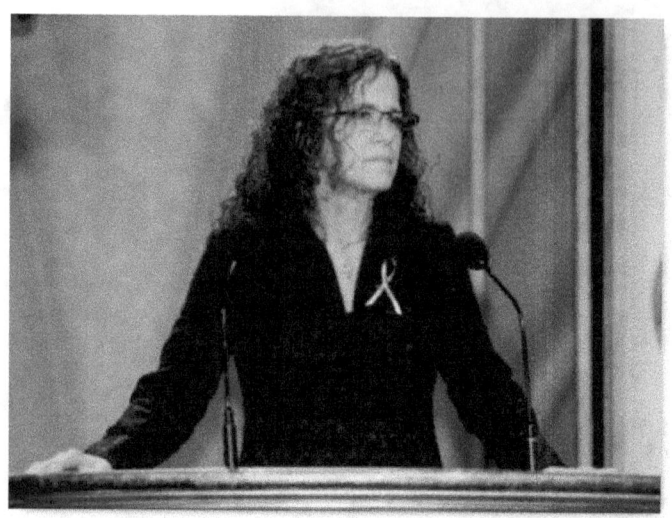

Genita M. Mason H.H.P., N.C., M.H.
Medical Director The Biosanctuary
2010 Recipient of the CCHR Human Rights Award
& The 2014 American Board of Naturopathic
Medicine's High Achievement Award

"It is with deep gratitude that I accept this award from CCHR and I thank you for the countless lives you have saved through your passion and dedication to such a noble cause. Not one of us should have to settle for what psychiatry is offering - misinformation, false labels and lethal drugs which do nothing - but destroy the body and mind. Our children deserve better. Our friends and family deserve better. Humanity deserves better.

The unholy alliance between the pharmaceutical and psychiatric industries presents a pseudo medical model that inflicts addictive, chemical abuse on millions of innocent victims under the guise of medicine. Well isn't it time we said, "ENOUGH"? Isn't it time we started demanding that our governments stop funding this pseudoscience, this grim fairy tale called psychiatry?

—

Just examine their statistics - billions of dollars in funding yet they have no cures, no successes. Only victims. It is time for a new model of mental health care to emerge. One with respect for the body and the mind and compassion for those in distress. One that treats patients with respect and with dignity. One that has proven success, one that actually cures. That model is Green Mental Health Care.

We need to spread the word; there is a non-toxic, non-invasive and non-addictive solution for mental health issues. And we must - all of us - REFUSE to settle for less. You are all healers and you are all heroes.

Thank you."
Genita M. Mason H.H.P., N..C., M.H.

Green Mental Health Care

How to Get Off
&
Stay Off Psychiatric Drugs

A Non-Toxic, Non-Invasive, Non-Addictive Approach

Staying Sane in a Toxic World

Genita M. Mason H.H.P., N.C., M.H. Medical Director, The Biosanctuary
A Green Body & Mind Medical Model Practicing High Impact Biological Medicine for Orthomolecular Neurochemical Rehabilitation
www.thebiosanctuary.com US: (877) 285.9266

Table of Contents

—

—

—

Introduction

What is Green Mental HealthCare?

Green Mental Health Care is based on the preservation and treatment of the mind and body (for they are not separate functions) using non-toxic, non-addictive, and non-invasive strategies that produces good mental health. Green Mental Health Care has not only proven to be superior in patient outcomes than any other treatment method, including the use of psychiatric drugs, but it achieves the patient's health goals at a fraction of the cost while saving them from the life-threatening health risks associated with psychiatric drugs.

The Green Mental Health movement recognizes that the #1 cause of today's mental health problems—from depression, anxiety, "ADHD," "Bi-Polar Disorder" to even "Schizophrenia"—are the result of exposure to and accumulation of toxins that destroy the body's natural ability to function with particular focus on how this effects someone's mental and emotional well-being.

The Green Mental Health movement employs real medical diagnostics and non- toxic, non-addictive, non-invasive, non-harmful medical solutions. It does not rely on pseudoscience or "chemical imbalance" theories of the brain that have never been scientifically/medically proven to exist or the administration of drugs that are toxic in the truest sense of the word, as psychiatric drugs actually destroy cells and tissue.

To clear up the "chemical imbalance" controversy, psychiatry and the pharmaceutical companies are pushing the idea that you have an inherent chemical imbalance in the brain and they have a pill that will correct it. This is not true!

They have created this fairy tale based on pseudoscience to sell their products. This claim that is void of any proof or scientific explanation implies that there is something inherently wrong with you and nothing could be farther from the truth. Your brain is doing exactly what it is supposed to be doing; it is reporting that there is something wrong in the body. The brain is a very dense collection of endocrine glands and nerves. The nerves read the internal and external environmental factors and call upon the endocrine glands (hypothalamus, pituitary, pineal, thyroid, parathyroid, adrenals, testes, ovaries, and pancreas) to provide the chemicals required to survive (adapt) to the environment the organism (you) lives in. When the environment is nutritionally deficient or physically threatening, the glands become fatigued or deficient and become unable to respond appropriately to the requests of the nervous system. The chemicals they are supposed to provide are no longer made available which throws the entire body out of balance (homeostasis) and the brain reports this. So yes, there is a chemical imbalance due to a damaged or deficient organ but it is not a genetic or inherent condition. It is entirely correctable by healing the organ that is deficient so that it produces the chemicals nature has relied on it to do for millions of years to maintain homeostasis in the human body. For instance, those with poor diets, sedentary lifestyles and stressful jobs and home lives tend to develop adrenal fatigue.

This is when your adrenals begin failing in producing enough cortisol to mediate stress in your life. This condition is well known to cause anxiety, nervousness, anxiousness, hyper-reactivity, emotional outbursts and even panic attacks because you don't have enough cortisol going to the brain to balance out the over stimuli caused by demands of your lifestyle. Now is the root cause of your symptoms in your head? No. So I guess in a round a about way it could be viewed as a chemical imbalance because you are low on cortisol but this is not how psychiatry is following through with the message that you have a chemical imbalance in your brain. They don't look for the root cause and correct it—they give you a pill that actually does more damage to the body and mind. As a result, because they are very potent endocrine disruptors (creating widespread hormonal imbalance), they create extreme real chemical imbalances because they are toxic chemicals that do not belong in the body. In fact, they harm every organ in the body making them deficient and unable to produce the chemicals required for the body and brain to operate in the way they are designed to. There is no inherent "chemical imbalance". There is a deficiency due to a malfunctioning or damaged organ and the good news is, is that you can not only find the root cause of the problem by going to a real doctor that uses diagnostics to establish what is wrong with your health, but also choose from a long list of healthy, non-toxic and non-addictive ways heal and become whole and vibrant again. The solutions become evident once the real problem is exposed!

With millions upon millions taking toxic psychiatric drugs, we must ask the fundamental question: how did we get here? The answer is simple. We've been brainwashed by a multi-billion dollar mental health industry's marketing campaign. We've bought into psychiatrists repackaging behaviors as mental "diseases." We've been inundated with drug commercials about chemical imbalances and the "wonder drugs" to treat them. The media has continually promoted psychiatrists conducting studies that supposedly show the efficacy and safety of the latest greatest psychiatric drug—never bothering to find out that these psychiatrists are paid mouthpieces for the psycho/pharmaceutical industry. The government has bought into mental health "patient's rights groups" frantically lobbying for more drugs and more drug treatment on behalf of the "mentally ill" when in fact these groups are also on Big Pharma's payroll.

Their heavily funded marketing strategy worked and is reflected in the different standards we hold mainstream medical doctors to, as opposed to psychiatrists. For example, if the average person experienced some physical discomfort for which they had no explanation, they would go to a medical doctor to find out what was causing it. Now imagine if this person walked into his doctors office, complaining about this discomfort, the doctor proceeded to ask him a few questions, writing down a few notes, then proclaimed, "You have cancer and will need chemotherapy." No blood tests, X-Rays or lab tests to prove it—just a medical diagnoses requiring medical intervention—based simply on questions, not lab tests. Would the average person buy it? Of course not.

Well why is it different with a mental health diagnoses? Why do we believe a psychiatrist or any doctor could determine we are "mentally ill" or have a "chemical imbalance" requiring the administration of a powerful and mind-altering drug with absolutely no medical evidence to back them up?

Because we've been sold a bill of goods, which is actually a very misleading and dangerous bill of not so goods.

Few people realize that depression, anxiety, behavioral problems and even psychosis are nearly always the result of an undiagnosed medical condition. And by medical condition I mean something that can be confirmed medically to exist, with medical tests.

For example, depression is frequently caused by low thyroid function; anxiety can be caused by low adrenal function; extreme mood swings can be caused by hypoglycemia1 or low blood sugar. And these are simply a few of the more common causes (more on this later in the brochure).

The point is that 99.5% of all mental health issues can be directly traced to a malfunctioning organ, typically of the neuroendocrine2 system—your pharmacist within.

---

1 Hypoglycemia: abnormal decrease of sugar in the blood.
2 Neuroendocrine: of, relating to, or involving the hormonal substance that influences the nervous system.

Chapter One

The Toxic Environment

Today's very toxic world is the number one cause of mental health problems that people suffer. Everything is toxic today; our food, air, water, soil, home cleaning and personal hygiene products, lawn and garden care, even Mr. Bubble! Unfortunately, now the "medicine" (drugs) to "cure" people's mental problems are in fact the most dangerous toxic chemicals of all—resulting in hundreds of thousands of deaths per year in the U.S. alone.

So when someone is given psychiatric drugs they are simply adding more toxic chemicals to what is in all likelihood, an already toxic body whose mind is symptomatic because of it!

In the U.S. alone, there are over 100,000 toxic chemicals released into our air, food, water and soil. Most of the toxins are brain and endocrine system disrupters and accumulate in the system causing cross contamination toxicities. The body and mind are being assaulted daily by these life- and presence-of-mind robbing agents and unfortunately when the symptoms from their damage present themselves, instead of finding out what is causing the problem, they are further victimized by toxic "medicine" that aggravates the root cause of the symptoms and places the person in even graver health risk danger.

Since the majority of all toxins cause brain and endocrine damage, resulting in adverse mental health symptoms, I'm sure you realize that this builds a strong case for Green Mental Health. Toxic chemicals are directly linked to negatively affecting these body functions:

- Our immune system
- Our endocrine system
- Our nervous system
- Our reproductive system

As an example of toxins in our environment, a study conducted by the Environmental Working Group sheds light on the extent of toxins in our environment:

A study conducted on newborns by the Environmental Working Group (EWG) found an average of 200 industrial chemicals and pollutants in umbilical cord blood from 10 babies born in August and September of 2004 in U.S. hospitals. Tests revealed a total of 287 chemicals in the group. The umbilical cord blood of these 10 children, collected by Red Cross after the cord was cut, contained pesticides, consumer product ingredients, and wastes from burning coal, gasoline, and garbage.

Of the 287 chemicals detected in umbilical cord blood, 180 cause cancer in humans and animals, 217 are toxic to the brain and nervous system, and 208 cause birth defects or abnormal development in animal tests. The dangers of pre- or post-natal exposure to this complex mixture of carcinogens, developmental toxins and neurotoxins have never been studied.3

3

http://www.ewg.org/reports/bodyburden2/execsumm.php

Chapter Two

What Are Neurotoxins?

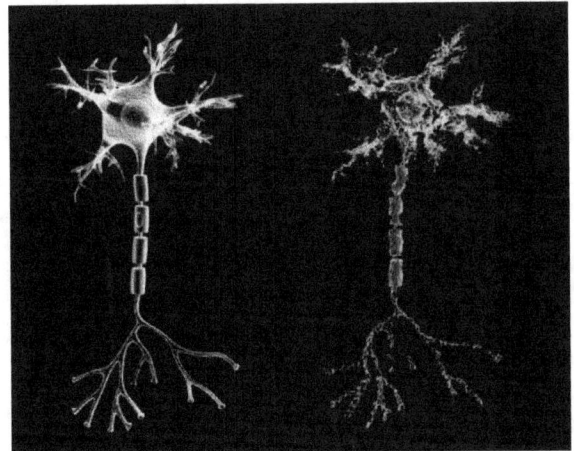

Healthy Cell   Cell damaged by neurotoxicity

Neurotoxins are chemicals that are toxic to the body.
Neurotoxic effectively means "nerve poison." It means the
poison's chemical structure damages the cellular structures
of neurons and the central nervous system. The following
are examples of neurotoxins or things that can be neurotoxic
when taken in excess:

- Psychiatric drugs (psychiatric drugs are actually more
  dangerous than most illicit drugs because they are
  synthetic and cannot be broken down by the body.
  This is not to condone street drugs, but to put into
  perspective just how damaging psychiatric drugs are)
- Illicit Drugs
- Pesticides (abundant in commercially grown foods,
  personal hygiene and many other products)

- Lawn and garden pesticides, insecticides and herbicides
- Sugar substitutes (Aspartame, NutraSweet, Splenda, Equal, etc.)
- Home cleaning chemicals
- Carbon monoxide from car exhaust
- Heavy metals such as mercury, (main sources are vaccinations, fish, and amalgam [silver fillings]), lead and aluminum
- Many food additives (chemicals) used in processed foods
- Excess natural and processed sugars (over stimulates and then kills brain cells—also "suffocates" cells so that nutrients can't get in and toxins can't get out, resulting in cell death)
- Tobacco (most of the over 500 chemicals used in tobacco)
- Excess conventional dairy and grains (clogs cells causing waste build up which advances cell death)
- Toxic saturated fats found in animal meats due to drugs and hormones they are chemically abused with
- Excess stimulants such as coffee, tea and energy drinks
- Many body lotions, deodorants, and other neurotoxic products such as Mr. Bubble
- Industrial pollution
- Genetically modified foods

As each of us has different immune systems, and different chemical sensitivities, it is understandable that not all of us will experience severe mental duress or the symptoms of mental "illness" due to exposure to these neurotoxic agents. They are not good for any of us, but some will be more adversely affected than others. The point is that all of the above items can cause loss of mental health and can result in anxiety, depression, mood swings, hyperactivity, inability to focus or retain information, hyper-reactivity, explosive moods up and down, obsessive characteristics, compulsiveness, forgetfulness, paranoia, fear, worry—each and every "condition" psychiatrists prescribe very toxic drugs for. In fact, the lion's share of the cause of addictive biochemistry4 which leads to drug and/or alcohol addiction is a direct result of one attempting to self-medicate the symptoms created by the accumulative damage being done by any one or a combination of the list above.

Depending on your inherent chemical sensitivities, general lifestyle, dietary habits and health of your liver which is loaded down with the responsibility to attempt to detoxify these brain and nervous system damaging agents, your level of poisoning will adversely affect you resulting in each and every one of the symptoms psychiatrists are labeling as mental disorders such as anxiety, fatigue, bipolar, depression, schizophrenia, OCD, ADD/HD, social phobias and sadly the list goes on and gets larger every year. In addition, we all have different food sensitivities, and many people do not know that food allergies can cause many symptoms of mental illness. Often food allergies are a direct result of the liver being sluggish from years of neuro- and other toxic chemical abuse including psychiatric drugs.

Neurotoxins also damage and kill neurons because they cause seriously accelerated oxidative stress. Oxidative stress is also known as free radical5 damage. Both refer to how cells are damaged by an over abundance of oxidants in the body. Oxidants are oxygen molecules6 that "steal" electrons from cells making them unable to function. A good example of this is your windshield wipers: they become brittle, crack and deteriorate due to the "cross linking" with oxygen molecules. It's quite easy to replace your windshield wipers; the same isn't so for your brain. If there are not enough anti-oxidants in the system to replace the electrons that oxidants steal, they will cause a cascade reaction that erodes the cell and causes first cellular death, then death of larger groups, or legions of tissues which will interfere with the functioning of the organ itself—enter mental health symptoms.

It's also important to note that it is not just the neurotoxins in our vaccines (mercury, aluminum), food (pesticides, MSG, Aspartame and hundreds of others), air, water, homes, schools, lawns and psychiatric drugs that are deteriorating the mental health of people but also the excessive caffeine and sugar which over stimulate the sympathetic nervous system7 causing anxiety, low blood sugar issues (hypoglycemia), insomnia, depression, and each and every one of the conditions mentioned throughout this pamphlet. So, when faced with adverse mental health symptoms, why not instead of adding to the problem risking disease, death and certainly diminishing quality of life, take the toxin out rather than adding to them with psychiatric drugs?

---

4 Biochemistry: the study of chemical processes in living organisms.

5 Free radical: a destructive molecule. A group of atoms that has one or more unpaired electrons that causes them to be very chemically reactive. In the body, free radicals are produced by natural biological processes or introduced from the environment (as in tobacco smoke, toxins, pollutants, etc.), which can damage one's cells, proteins, and DNA by altering their chemical structure.

One of the most important things to know in today's world of sales science and criminal misinformation is that while yes, these neurotoxic poisons do damage the brain and nervous system which is causing the epidemic mental health crisis we are experiencing, they also damage every other critical organ and greater than 95% of the time it is the failing of one of these organs such as the adrenals, thyroid, liver, pancreas and stomach/intestines that is the root cause of the adverse mental symptoms people suffer—from depression and anxiety to bipolar and schizophrenia. There is a physical underlying root cause. Always. When people become "symptomatic," meaning they exhibit signs of stress, worsening mood, depression, it is because their body is trying to tell them something is not functioning right.

6 Molecule: the smallest particle of a substance that retains all the properties of the substance and is composed of one or more atoms.

7 Sympathetic Nervous System: the part of the autonomic nervous system originating in the middle and lower regions of the spinal cord that generally reduce digestive secretions, speed up the heart and contract blood vessels. Notably used in the body's "flight or fight" system

Chapter 3

How Psych Drugs Are Neurotoxic

Because psychiatric drugs are developed to affect neurochemistry8 they are "built" to specifically manipulate the function of neurons in the brain and nervous system. And just like all other neurotoxins, they are known to be "endocrine disruptors" which adversely affects hormonal balance.

From the very first dose, psychiatric drugs begin damaging the mitochondria of cells. The mitochondria is the energy production plant for the cell which uses carbohydrates to make energy for the cell to do what it is designed to do, repair and replicate. As the mitochondria becomes "sick" or sluggish, it is unable to create the energy that the cell requires to function and this results in the body (and brain) going into toxic overload because the cell doesn't have the energy to detoxify or get the waste out. The liver becomes sluggish and toxins begin to recirculate throughout the body. When the mitochondria of cells become damaged there is no limit on what kind of disease or mental symptom can develop as each and every cell of the body relies on the mitochondria for healthy functioning. Mitochondrial9 damage results in "side effects" (which are really direct effects), and the plethora of diseases psychiatric drugs are linked to from diabetes to cancer. A large part of the reason that psychiatric drugs cause weight gain is due to the mitochondria's progressive inability to properly convert carbohydrates and fats to energy.

Psychiatric drugs literally chew away at brain cells until they completely disintegrate and their protein breakdown by-products are ingested by the system.

Accumulation in the body of the waste products of neurotoxic destruction of brain cells is one condition that leads to Alzheimer's and Parkinson's disease, as does the toxic agent that is causing the brain cell death. The gradual build up of the drug combined with the body's diminishing ability to get it out of the system wreak havoc on cellular functions and set the stage for the many, many diseases psychiatric drugs are known to cause (heart attack, stroke, sudden death, liver disease, tics, involuntary muscle spasms, stunted growth, diabetes, etc).

---

[8] **Neurochemistry:** the study of the chemical structure and processes of the nervous system and the effects of chemicals on it.

[9] **Mitochondrial:** of or relating to mitochondria. Mitochondria are a specific part within cells that act as the cell's power-plant, they make and supply energy to the cells.

For a current listing of the side (direct) effects and how lethal psychiatric drugs are, consider the documented side effects of these commonly prescribed psychiatric drugs by international drug regulatory agencies at: http://www.cchrint.org/psychdrugdangers/

Also be sure to download the free brochure, *The Side Effects of Common Psychiatric Drugs.*

How Psychiatric Drugs Cause Addiction

There is another very dangerous activity going on: because the body needs to make biochemical changes to accommodate the drug, neurochemical adaptation, better known as addiction, occurs. Psychiatric drugs are synthetic and made purposely to not break down easily in the system. This is why such a small amount goes a long way. This is not good because it causes the body and mind to develop a deeper relationship, or dependence on the drug, and because the half life is 5 to 10 times longer, the drug has more time with and access to the cells to damage them. These synthetic drugs are designed to replace or alter (increase or decrease) your body's natural production of the neurochemicals it needs to function—this is a true chemical imbalance because it ignores or bypasses the brain's mechanisms for balance or "homeostasis." When the body and brain are healthy they can create the exact amounts of what they need in neurotransmitters and hormones by using a feedback system which tells them there is enough and they will slow down production of the chemical, or if there is too much, reduce receptor sites to maintain balance. However, in the case of drugs, the feedback system will try and reduce it via enzymatic ingestion but can't, so then it will reduce its own production of the neurochemical the drug is mimicking as well as the receptors for that drug which puts the person in grave danger should they lose their bottle of pills on the wrong day!

The end result is not only a strong dependence on the drug but the desire to avoid the symptoms from the damage they have caused, which creates an even greater psychological dependence.

And finally, neurotoxins mutate genes and genetic expression and interfere with fetal development. There is no mystery as to why birth defects have skyrocketed in the last 30 years since Big Pharma has been saturating the public and practitioners with claims made only by their own pseudoscience that they have answers for mental health issues. The opposite is true. They are actually a part of the problem of the growing epidemic mental health issues today. Doesn't it make sense that if they had solutions, the reported mental health complaints would decrease? So why are mental health issues growing yearly?

Psychiatric drugs are neurotoxic chemicals designed to "kill the messenger" of bad news—what is left of brain function slowly deteriorates and becomes symptomatic and this is why people are given multiple diagnosis over time. Every organ of the body required for good mental health is compromised by these neurotoxins and there is no avoiding the damage they are known to inflict while on them. People are getting sicker and sicker because they are not addressing the root cause of their symptoms, but instead are taking toxic drugs that only add to the original health issue while causing their own.

Chapter 4
What's Causing People's Mental Symptoms?

When you get a pain in your side your brain reports the pain but you realize that it is a muscle cramp or gas that is causing the pain. You realize that it is not your brain causing the pain. People don't realize that their mental health symptoms do not originate in their brain—the brain is simply the messenger. Your body is trying to save your life by letting you know something in your body is going wrong. Your brain is working right. It is doing what it is supposed to do—report the problem.Your brain is the reporting system for your internal and external environment. It is not your brain's fault that it is cold outside and you are uncomfortable without adequate clothing, no more than it is your brain's fault that you are experiencing anxiety in response to the damage your adrenals are suffering due to excess coffee or other nervous system stimulants over-stimulating you. It is not your brain's fault that it is not getting all the raw materials in the way of nutrients it needs to produce the neurotransmitters and hormones it requires for good health and to help you get through life's common emotional and psychological challenges such as the loss of a job or loved one causing you to sink into chronic depression. So many people enter crisis today in such marginal mental and physical shape that it is nearly impossible for them to climb out of adverse emotional and psychological strains they suffer. Your brain relies on the healthy functioning of each and every organ of your body to provide you mental health in good times and bad, so you must take care of the whole body to achieve Green Mental Health.

How Neurotoxins Cause Adverse Mental Health Symptoms

Neurotoxins target brain cells and they do most of their

damage within the brain and nervous system. However, that damage is also known to cause endocrine or hormonal issues that also serve up many of today's adverse mental health symptoms.

Neurotoxins shrink vital glands and centers within the brain such as the hypothalamus and the pituitary.

Neurotoxins cause mitochondria damage10. This will have a deleterious effect on the entire body and mind since the mitochondria supplies the energy for the cell. Reduce the energy and you reduce the functional capacity of the cell to utilize nutrients and remove waste. This will cause advanced oxidative stress thus damage to those organs affected the most which is usually the organs the drugs are manufactured to affect, the brain and nervous system thus disrupting the entire endocrine system as well.

----

[10] Medication-induced mitochondrial damage and disease John Neustadt and Steve R. Pieczenik.

What Can Cause Panic Attacks, Mood Swings and Depression

To give an extremely simple broad example of how the physical malfunctioning of an organ can cause adverse mental health symptoms: the hypothalamus produces a hormone called Corticotrophin Releasing Hormone (CRH) that stimulates the pituitary to produce another hormone, Adrenocorticotropic (ACTH). This hormone stimulates release of Cortisol, your stress buffer hormone, from the adrenals. If the hypothalamus, pituitary or adrenals are fatigued, under toxic assault, malnourished or damaged then you will have little to no stress buffer being produced in your body to maintain homeostasis in the brain during periods of time that it would require it. Loss of homeostasis or balance due to low cortisol levels will produce mental health symptoms such as irritation, increased perception of stress, anxiety, panic, paranoia, depression, nervousness, and fatigue. Depending on blood sugar regulation and the person's propensity to experience low blood sugar episodes this condition could also cause the person to experience extreme mood swings and emotional outbursts. That is just one very simplified example and remember that this a physical cause of mental health symptoms.

It is important to note here that neurotoxic drugs such as psychiatric drugs are endocrine disruptors and disrupt the body's blood sugar regulation mechanisms. This should give a good fundamental understanding as to why in many cases psychiatric drugs actually intensify symptoms the patient is trying to medicate as well as cause new ones.

What Can Cause Anxiety, Depression And Bipolar

The pituitary releases the thyroid hormone, TSH which regulates thyroid function. When this hormone goes high it indicates that the thyroid is producing low thyroid hormone which can set a cascade of symptoms and conditions in motion from depression and bipolar to headaches, irritability[11]and anxiety. Note that all of these are perceived to be "in your head" but they are not. They originated due to low thyroid hormone output.

Scientists now consider thyroid hormone (TH) one of the major "players" in brain chemistry disorders. And as with any brain chemical disorder, until treated correctly, thyroid hormone imbalance has serious effects on the patient's emotions and behavior.[12]

TH acts as a neurotransmitter. TH imbalance can mimic psychiatric disease because TH influences levels of serotonin, a neurotransmitter integral to moods and behavior. Low levels of TH can cause depression. Some anti-depressants make hypothyroid patients feel even worse because the medications depress TH levels. Paradoxically, some substances labeled depressants such as alcohol or opiates can increase TH levels by impairing the breakdown of TH in the brain, thus lifting mood. This may be one reason why these substances are so addictive.

---

[11] DeGroot, The Thyroid and Its Diseases, 1996

[12] Dr. Ridha Arem, *The Thyroid Solution: A Mind Body Program for Beating Depression and Regaining Your Emotional and Physical Healt*

What Can Cause Psychosis / Schizophrenia

There are many biochemical factors that can cause psychosis/schizophrenia. From food allergies and chemical sensitivities to toxic exposures. However, one biochemical process that needs more attention because it affects so many people is the adrenochrome connection established by Dr. Abram Hoffer.

Adrenochrome is a toxic hormone made in the body by the oxidation (meaning breakdown) of adrenaline. Adrenochrome can be converted into either of two other compounds: dihydroxyindole or adrenolutin. It is possible that dihydroxyindole balances off adrenaline to reduce tension and irritability. In schizophrenics, however, adrenochrome is converted primarily into adrenolutin, which is toxic, and the combination of adrenochrome-adrenolutin results in a toxic assault on brain.

Adrenochrome is a hallucinogenic and is linked to the aural and visual hallucinations that many schizophrenics experience. Those who produce too much adrenochrome do so because their bodies don't metabolize adrenaline into its harmless by-products efficiently and instead it is oxidized and converts into adrenochrome.

Two factors are common in the production of adrenochrome that can be corrected in the victims of this disruptive biochemical pathway; an overload of adrenaline combined with oxidative stress. This is why Dr. Abram Hoffer's niacin and vitamin C therapy, along with other considerations the patient required, was so effective.

What defines an "overload of adrenaline" is dependent on each individual. Meaning that different people have different capacities for safely clearing adrenaline from the system depending on their stores of those nutrients required to do so and the absence of hyper oxidation. Those individuals that responded well to this treatment did so because the niacin reduces adrenaline release and vitamin C, being an anti- oxidant, reduces the oxidative stress on the body—in combination they work to reduce adrenochrome.

There are thousands of neurotoxins including psychiatric drugs that can induce the adrenochrome internally made chemical cocktail and this can be one of the underlying mechanisms of action that produces the suicidal and homicidal ideation that many people on psychiatric drugs experience as they are one of the most potent and common neurotoxins causing oxidative stress in humans today.

What Can Cause Hyperactivity, ADHD, OCD, etc.

When we consider how many children experience hyperactiviy, over-excitability, the inability to focus, and emotional hyper-reactivity or absolute mental lethargy, one has to ask, "why are so many children affected with these conditions when 70 years ago it was extremely rare?" Researching how few references there are of these issues in children in medical reviews of the early 1900's can substantiate this.

The answer to that would be in the question "What has changed the most affecting the lives of children over the last 70 years?" Food and the chemicals they are putting on and in it and of course sugars and stimulants.

———

It is established that the soil today is now over 80% deficient in the minerals we require for healthy minds and bodies. That is not good when you consider that the famous scientist and double Nobel Prize Laureate (peace and chemistry) Linus Pauling stated, "One could trace every disease and every ailment to a mineral deficiency." This includes symptoms that classify as mental health issues. No pun intended, but minerals are the bedrock of human nutrition. Vitamin literally means "vital mineral". Our food chain is poisoning us and children are the most symptomatic because their detoxification systems are not mature enough to win the fight against the over 3,000 toxic chemicals they are exposed to even before birth, many of which compromise the health of their neuroendocrine system before they are even born.

Heavy metal toxicity is becoming more and more epidemic today along side the mental health disorders they cause. Amalgam dental fillings, thimerosal (mercury) in vaccinations, fish, pesticides, fungicides and insecticides are the most potent sources of mercury poisoning today. Lead, mercury, antimony, arsenic are all established to cause mental health issues including ADD/HD, autism, mental lethargy, etc. Think about it—metals are conductors! And that is exactly what they do, stimulate conductivity throughout the body and over stimulate everything from mental to physical nerve communication processes—and when you over stimulate you cause advanced cell death!

These topics are exposed in far greater detail in the full book but to counter the biggest lie on the airwaves which the pharmaceutical and sugar industries own with their advertising dollars I will demonstrate with real science of how sugar over stimulates a child and then make it impossible for them to relax and learn something. To begin this example, I will start with this: Think about the last time you nearly escaped a car accident, remember how your pulse was raised, your heart was pounding and your thoughts were distant yet at the same time all over the map. How feasible would it have been in that moment to sit down and study for a college final? Or prepare a report for work?

Or learn a new, second language? Well, that is exactly the same biochemistry playing itself out in a child on a high simple carbohydrate; cereal, bread, pasta, candy, coke, and other processed foods— sugary dead-food diet. And you can rest assured that if the child's diet is not designed to avoid refined sugar, it is most likely filled with aspartame—other toxic sweeteners, stimulants and chemical food additives that will ensure a lifetime of physical and mental symptoms robbing them of quality of life, opportunity and peace of mind.

Excess sugar in the diet will cause a spike in insulin that in turn will drive sugar levels to abnormal lows. This will cause a release of adrenaline to stimulate glycogen release from the liver. The added energy from the glycogen release combined with the adrenaline is the simplified explanation of how sugar creates hyperactivity, agitation, and the inability to focus in children. Over time, the adrenals will become fatigued (I have tested children as young as 4 years old positive for adrenal exhaustion!) and when the resulting low cortisol effects on the brain are combined with the low blood sugar symptoms children can become irritable, hyper emotional (temper tantrums), destructive, angry and even violent.

The blood sugar roller coaster these diets produce also burn out the thyroid and cause mental health issues involving low Thyroid Hormone.

When considering all the other toxic assaults children endure which the lion's share are extremely neurotoxic, there is no question as to where the root cause of this epidemic of mental distress and symptoms of over stimulation—then complete mental and physical exhaustion in both children and adults originates.

The blood sugar roller coaster exhausts every gland and function of the neuroendocrine system that can and does create all the common mental health complaints today. Sugar is the real gateway drug because it sets the person up for a lifetime of symptoms that they will seek to self medicate any way they can. Addictive biochemistry—such as a predisposition for alcohol addiction is many times established by the over consumption of sugar at a young age. This can cause such sugar dysregulation issues that the chronic highs and especially low blood sugar symptoms (including those of the low TH which usually accompanies this condition) will create a clear path to alcohol as a "medicine" for the symptoms they suffer.

Researchers at Mt. Sinai School of Medicine studied 163 men and women who had no personal history of alcoholism or other drug use. Half of the participants had a family history of alcoholism, while the other half did not.

The researchers found that study participants with a family history of alcoholism were 2.5 times more likely to have a sweet tooth compared to the other group.13

A family history of alcoholism would indicate the child was born of a family line with a deficient neuroendocrine system most likely caused by alcohol and other dietary and lifestyle behaviors that would damage the body's sugar regulation systems. This does not indicate that there is a genetic disposition; it indicates there is an inherent disposition that can be corrected with dietary and lifestyle modifications that serve to heal those damaged organs of the neuroendocrine system.

Another gateway to accelerated brain cell death and over stimulation is the fact that neurotoxins such as psych drugs and mercury eat away at the membranes of cells. This reduces the cells protective coating, which "chooses" what goes in and out of the cell. When this membrane is damaged, it can cause an over firing between cells which over stimulates the person and causes symptoms such as anxiety and hyperactivity.

13
http://www.cheersbook.com/who/The_Council_on_Alcohol_and_Drugs_News_Today.html

Candida, Parasites, Fungus, Leaky Gut, Bacterial Dysbiosis[14]

Many neurotoxins (mercury and psychiatric drugs being the most common) are at the root cause of Candida, viral and pathogenic infections. Neurotoxins are known to have an affinity to damage the mitochondria of the cell thus the cell's ability to process carbohydrates efficiently. When you don't process carbohydrates properly they ferment in the body and provide an ideal environment for unfriendly over-growths such as Candida (yeast), harmful bacteria, parasites, viruses, and fungus causing Bacterial Dysbiosis and Leaky Gut Syndrome among many other digestive abnormalities. Benzodiazepines, neurotoxins in the tranquilizer category of drugs, cause Leaky Gut syndrome and Bacterial Dysbiosis because they subdue the intestinal tract along with the rest of the body and mind, reducing stomach motility15 thus causing food to sit and decompose adding to an ideal yeast and bacterial environment. This of course also promotes an acidic system that is an ideal environment for yeast, fungi, virus, and even cancer.

Candida and other conditions caused by sugars fermenting in the body and bacterial overgrowths has long been linked to be the root cause in many individuals of chronic depression, mental and physical fatigue, hypoglycemia, anxiety, OCD, ADD/HD, and the list unfortunately goes on and on.

Negatively offsetting the gut flora16 can also result in serious digestive disorders, gas, irregular and unhealthy bowel movements and mild to sever malnutrition psychosis can develop.

———

Neurotoxins also cause the system to become acidic, which provides an ideal environment for yeast, bacterial, viral and fungal infections which can produce extremely adverse mental health reactions.

I have provided only a few of the hundreds of known biochemical processes associated with the deterioration of the organs of the body caused by neurotoxins that will produce adverse mental health symptoms.

---

[14] **Dysbiosis:** the condition of having microbial imbalances on or within the body. Dysbiosis is most prominent in the digestive tract or on the skin, but can also occur on any exposed surface or mucous membrane.

[15] **Motility:** moving or capable of moving spontaneously.

[16] **Gut flora:** the microorganisms that normally live in the digestive tracts of humans and other animal.

Do Not Stop Diagnostics Until You Are Presented with Evidence of the Root Cause!

The human experience today is chemically and energetically over stimulated and the body's adaptation and recovery methods simply cannot keep up. It is the neuroendocrine system, or the "pharmacist" within, that is charged with the job of adapting to the dietary and environmental "terrain" of life on the planet today and it is the pharmacist within that is becoming exhausted trying to keep up. Up until just a couple of hundred years ago, the body enjoyed the luxury of adapting to a natural environment that changed very slowly. Today, the body's adaptation center, the neuroendocrine system—your pharmacist within—is being taxed with the necessity of adapting to a world that has changed more in the last 100 years than in the last 500,000 years much of which is induced by toxic chemical assault. This applies to environmental toxicity, and the chemicals and loss of nutrition in our food when we need it the most as well as the energetic over stimulating aspects of modern living, which includes technology. Think about mail alone—we get more mail in one day than people typically got in a lifetime a hundred years ago!

The unfortunate thing is that when people experience intense mood swings, depression, insomnia, anxiety, attention problems, the very first thing they should look for is an underlying physical (not psychiatric) condition. People could save themselves so much loss of quality of life, time and money, as well as avoid the very real and common serious health risks associated with psychiatric drugs, if they simply found a healthcare practitioner that knows how the body and mind work together, is qualified to explore the condition, run lab tests for real diagnostics and then treat the underlying cause of their symptoms in a non-toxic, non-addictive an non-invasive way; the Green Way! This is the only real way to cure a mental health condition.

Underlying Medical Conditions That Can Manifest as Mental Health Problems

- Hypoadrenalism (Adrenal fatigue) – lowered cortisol levels. Cortisol is your stress buffer hormone and chronic stress will cause the adrenal glands to become fatigued. This can cause irritability, hyper-reactivity, moodiness, physical and mental fatigue, and a long list of other symptoms adversely affecting mental health.

- Hypothyroidism – which can cause low serotonin which is linked to depression

- Hypoglycemia – which can cause extreme mood swings generally labeled "bipolar". When hypoglycemia and adrenal fatigue are combined explosive highs and lows can be experienced and it is very common today directly as a result of excess sugars, caffeine and processed foods.

- Multiple Chemical Sensitivity (MCS) – which can cause each and every mental health complaint of today.

- Hypopituitarism – lowered secretion of vital hormones the rest of the endocrine system requires to regulate the body and mind.

- Deterioration of the general nervous system through chronic hyper stimulation of the sympathetic nervous system as a result of job / home / relationship stress or excess stimulants including those found in processed foods.

- Brain and nervous system damage as a result of aspartame. Many people have been diagnosed with multiple sclerosis and found later it was overall deterioration of the nervous system directly due this excitotoxin.

- Liver Disease – the liver is the hardest hit organ today trying to keep up with our toxic world.

- Candida (Yeast) infections – which cause a multitude of

adverse mental health symptoms from chronic depression to anxiety and even schizophrenia.

- Heart Disease.
- Developing brain cancer and aneurisms as a result of carcinogenic and neurotoxic chemicals.
- Digestive disorders furthering malnutrition that can even lead to malnutrition psychosis.
- Poor pancreatic function – which can cause nutritional deficiencies due to inadequate enzymes produced which causes mental symptoms and instability.
- A full spectrum of vitamin, mineral, essential fatty acids and enzyme deficiencies that can cause a plethora of adverse mental health conditions.

Note: There is a "hyper" for every "hypo" meaning that there is a chemical or condition which is causing excess hormones to be excreted from a gland such as too much insulin being poured into the system in response to chronic excess sugars in the diet or excess cortisol in response to chronic stress.

Each and every one of these and many we don't have the room to list, will cause nervousness, anxiety, depression, ADD/HD, hyperactivity, extreme mood swings, violent or hyper-reactive states, mental and emotional instability, notable personality changes, insomnia, Multiple Sclerosis symptoms, Parkinson's, Alzheimer's, neuropathy, etc. Essentially all the symptoms that develop from an over-stimulated, failing nervous system.

What Does Psychiatry Do Instead of Testing for the Underlying Cause of Your Mental Health Complaints?

Toxic load puts an enormous tax on your nutritional status, draining essential nutrients required for repair and replication of the cells and protection from oxidative stress / free radical damage. Your body's ability and efficiency to detox determines your state of health which is dependent on your nutritional status / verses toxic load! Prolonged poisoning "empties the tank" and this is when disease sets in. However, long before disease develops you will usually become symptomatic because of a combination of organs are beginning to fail. This is when it is time to listen to your body and the symptoms you are experiencing (which will many times be mental) and go to a health practitioner that is going to help you find the root cause of the symptoms and is not going to simply treat the symptom. This can be very dangerous especially in the case of psychiatry. This pseudo-medical model uses more neurotoxic drugs to mask the symptom which is like cutting the wire to the oil lamp in your car. The warning light goes out but you are still low on oil and if you don't put some oil in your car it is going to blow the engine and you are going to be left without the car—or in this case, a body!

It would be extremely scary to be born without a system that reports health issues the body is struggling with. You need to view your symptoms differently. They are your friends; they are trying to save your life by letting you know something is wrong. If you cut the wires of the brain that is reporting those symptoms all you have done is provide opportunity for an even more dangerous health robbing situation by adding a body and brain damaging toxin to the system while leaving the root cause undiscovered and untreated—and what's even scarier is that you will not "see the light" many times until it is life threatening.

Chapter 5
What Your Doctor/Healthcare Provider Should Be Looking For

Toxic Load. A full toxicology report should be run on you. Depending on where you live, your lifestyle, where you work and diet you could be a walking toxic chemical cocktail.

- Reduced hormonal output of your pituitary.
- Liver function: low or sluggish liver function results in toxic waste build up in the body and causes neurological damage / dysfunction of the brain resulting in many of today's mental health issues.
- Hypoglycemia – blood sugar dysregulation is the #1 cause of mood swings, what is diagnosed as bipolar, anxiety, insomnia, mental and physical fatigue, etc.
- Adrenal fatigue. The lion's share of adults and many children test positive for low adrenal function.
- Low thyroid function
- Candida, fungus, mold and bacteria infections.
- Allergies
- Heavy metals
- Krebs Cycle[17]
- Methylation[18] Cycle
- Neurochemistry
- Pyroluria[19]
- Excess adrenochrome if you are having psychotic episodes.
- Nutritional status – malnutrition psychosis is extremely common. Don't be fooled by a full belly of toxic, empty calories.

- Hormonal assay. And do not fall into the Bio-identical Hormone Therapy trap. Work with a practitioner that will help you heal your endocrine glands so they produce adequate levels of the various hormones for you.

---

[17] **Krebs Cycle:** one of a series of chemical reactions in which the body's cells metabolize glucose for energy.

[18] **Methylation:** Methylation is the chemical reactions that place a methyl group (a combination of one carbon atom and three hydrogen atoms) at a particular spot on one's DNA during development of the organism. Testing for DNA methylation is said to help improve diagnosis of certain maladies.

[19] **Pyroluria:** a relatively unknown blood disorder which is hypothesized to cause a deficiency of vitamin B6 and zinc in a person. Pyroluria has been said to cause anxiety, depression and withdrawal.

Chapter 6
Five Reasons Why You Don't Want to Get Started on Psychiatric Drugs

To get well you are going to have to discover the root cause of your symptoms and a "chemical imbalance" is not the root cause! The cumulative effects of neuro and other toxins in our food and environment is the number one cause of mental health issues today. So it doesn't make sense to go to a doctor to get more neurotoxins to get well. It won't happen.

So it simply makes no sense to go to a doctor to get yet more toxins to poison the body and mind with—it will add to your mental health problems and will erode the health of many other organs as well.

There are a lot of reasons why you don't want to even get started on psych drugs.

They are addictive and extremely hard to get off of due to the frightening and painful withdrawal symptoms they are known to produce when you try to detox from them. The extreme withdrawal symptoms are caused not only from the body trying to readapt to the absence of the drug, but the damage that they have done to each and every one of your organs and how they take natural biochemical processes hostage which directly affects your brain chemistry and function. This promises even more symptoms with increased severity you will have to manage yourself out of if you try and get off of them.

While you are on them, not only does the original root cause of your symptoms continue to manifest and become more serious as a threat to your health, but the neurotoxic nature of the drug and the oxidative stress they cause actually

---

accelerates the underlying health issue that caused the symptoms in the first place. This is what invariably gives the many diseases they are associated with opportunity to manifest. The root cause of your symptoms is never explored, exposed and treated appropriately so it continues to get worse.

They cause mitochondrial damage. The mitochondria is the power house of the   cell—the energy producer. It converts carbohydrates to energy. When it becomes damaged, all functions of the cell begin to deteriorate and biochemical systems fail thus causing symptoms and then diseases, which if untreated can cause death. What is very serious about this is because you are on drugs that prevent the body from reporting symptoms, you have no idea that disease is manifesting within you and if you do have side effects and complain, they will simply put you on yet another drug to silence that negative condition which can only manifest into a serious health issue.

The cost involved. The best medical models available: Orthomolecular Neurochemical Rehabilitation (ONR) applied to Functional Medicine and Nutritional Neurochemistry services and medical oversight to safely get you off of drugs with minimal transitional discomfort and provide the Green Mental Health strategy that best responds to your individual needs for full recovery is typically an out of pocket expense. This medical model and the lab tests, other diagnostics, and specialized treatments required to get you sane in the membrane again and feeling peace and joy within can be quite costly and insurance does not cover it!

They will pay to get you addicted, but will basically tell you you're on your own when you want to get off. Sometimes they will do everything in their power to keep you on them such as threaten commitment (you are a threat to yourself or others) and force you into hospitalization. They wouldn't know how to help you off with minimal transitional discomfort anyway. All they know is how to get you on the drug—it is intended that you stay on them for life so they really don't know how to help you off. Additionally, it is becoming more and more popular to deny other health services if you do not comply with "standards of care" and these days that is toxic drugs. Many people are being forced into psychiatric wards today if they refuse medication. The entire system is built to get you in it and kept there. It is not a curative model; it is a managed care, treatment for life model. A life that is shortened an average of 25 years due to the toxic nature of psychiatric drugs!

You can avoid all these costs in health, time, money and loss of quality of life while enduring the long list of side effects and risking the well known psychotic and deadly ones which can result in suicide and murder simply by dismissing the idea of using a toxic drug to address your mental health issues and following the steps below to create a Green Mental Health Strategy that addresses your individual requirements to heal and enjoy excellent mental health.

There are no shortcuts; the laws of health are not negotiable. You must find the right health practitioner that is qualified to explore and discover the root cause of your symptoms and provide you proof in the way of diagnostics. You want the concrete evidence that justifies their evidence-based non-toxic, non-addictive and non- invasive treatment strategy. And then you must follow that treatment strategy.

The very good news is that if you are not on psychiatric drugs you can many times completely avoid a health care practitioner by following the strategy I am going to provide you in this pamphlet.

First and foremost you have to look at what to take out of the body in order to begin the healing process. Most doctors on both sides of the fence will consider first what you should add to the body and this is not good—when you treat symptoms you will be treating them forever. Western Medical doctors will add Statins20 or cholesterol lowering drugs to their diseased heart patients, psychiatrists will add brain and liver damaging, neurotoxic drugs to mask ill mental health symptoms, and many holistic practitioners will add Vitamin C for a cold. None of these approaches address the root cause of your heart disease, mental distress, or cold. Statins are the number one drug prescribed in the

—

US and heart attacks are the number one cause of death. Prescribing toxic drugs for mental health issues only allows the root cause to continue to manifest while doing additional damage to the body and mind. Vitamin C will help clear the cold a bit faster but does not address strengthening your immune system to best avoid flues, and other colds throughout the year.

So the first thing you want to do is to take out of the body what could be potentially making it ill.

Since I can give you at least 10 different biochemical pathways for each of the popular mental health complaints such as anxiety, ADD/HD, depression, bipolar, etc., (which confirms the need for laboratory tests before treatment is defined) the best way to approach a mental health healing event is to first, take out all things known to deteriorate and strain mental health.

This is more commonly known as detoxification. 95% plus of today's mental health issues are a direct result of diet and lifestyle. And now more than ever because conventional foods are becoming more and more adulterated with chemicals that are neurotoxic, inflicting damage of the brain and nervous system and are toxic in many other ways inflicting same damage on the rest of your critical organs.

When the body and mind is being poisoned, stress and the standard challenges making it in today's world are perceived to be far greater than they actually are because you are being slowly physically and mentally poisoned and deficient and wake up feeling overwhelmed and unable to meet the day's responsibilities and fear, paranoia, anxiety, depression and worry can become chronic.

---

[20] **Statins:** a class of drugs used to lower cholesterol.

Chapter 7
What to Do If You Are Symptomatic and Not on Psychiatric Drugs

A Green Mental Health Strategy starts with what to take out of your body!

Food additives such as preservatives, colorings, Aspartame, MSG, hydrogenated fats, essentially all chemicals used in food processing. These products are excito- neurotoxins, and carcinogenic which over stimulate and poison you, causing everything from depression and anxiety to seizures, aneurisms and cancer. Over- stimulated and symptomatic people are suffering and are toxic to the people in their immediate environment, which has a domino effect. These chemicals are toxic to all living organisms they come in contact with.

All sugar substitutes except Stevia—including Xylitol—have adverse health effects being reported from users. NutraSweet, Equal, Aspartame are all excito/neurotoxins and are likely to be causing the lions share of today's many neurological degenerative diseases including mental health decline and multiple sclerosis symptoms. Aspartame which is in the lion's share of sugar substitutes is made by Monsanto. Monsanto products have destroyed more earth, human and other life than possibly any other company. Their products include chemical warfare agents (Agent Orange), industrial materials (PCBs), food additives (NutraSweet), agrochemicals such as extremely toxic pesticides, herbicides, fungicides and insecticides that are all neurotoxins, and of course they make the crown of the crown of neurotoxins, pharmaceuticals. Not only do you not want the disease causing and deathly effects of their products in your home, food and "medicine", but also through purchasing their products you are empowering their pharmaceutical wing to control and manipulate the FDA and Congress. It is pretty much accepted as fact that Wall Street runs Congress now, so we've got to run Wall Street and you do that every time you spend your money. It is questionable if your vote matters every four years these days. Make sure your vote matters by using your dollars to vote and purchase only products made from companies that are not destroying the planet and especially in the case of pharmaceutical companies using their wealth to control your medical choices and even take your freedoms away such as in the case of forced drugging! We put them in power by using their products we can disempower them by discontinuing use of their products. In fact, this may be the only way we have left; it seems like just about everyone is paid off by them. And make no mistake; a big reason why your news is skewed in favor of their products is because the lights are on at every TV and radio station because of their advertising dollars.

Alcohol. Simply because it has no place in a detoxification process or a mental health crisis. Once your symptoms are cleared, and only if you do not have a problem with it, you may enjoy it occasionally.

Tobacco. If you're not ready to quit, switch to organic cigarettes such as American Spirits. Conventional cigarettes have over 500 other chemicals in them besides nicotine; the majority being neurotoxic. Please visit:

http://wiki.answers.com/Q/What_chemicals_are_in_cigarett es

And visit this link on smoking and mental health:
http://old.ash.org.uk/html/factsheets/html/fact15.html
The chemicals used in conventional cigarettes spread their toxicity every place a butt lands or the smoke reaches. Discontinuance of the rampant killer will help save your life and the life of the planet.

All caffeinated coffees and teas—including green tea. Caffeine, MSG and sugar substitutes are at the top of the list of the stimulants that are driving people crazy today robbing them of their peace of mind and everyone's around them.

Eliminating the toxic actions of those suffering these over stimulating, neurotoxic agents Greens up the community!

Sugars—all of them for at least two months—even the rich man's diabetes causing products such as agave, honey, fructose powder, etc. After that period of time you can enjoy natural sweeteners such as organic agave, yucon, and honey. Sugar is yet another factor greatly contributing to mental health problems. The natural ones must be used in moderation at very low quantities!

Pesticides. These very harmful and neurotoxic products are found in your food, water, personal hygiene products and on your lawns. Do not for a second under estimate the neurotoxic effects of pesticides especially on children. They cause brain cell death and damage to the nervous system causing hyperactivity, inability to focus, learning disabilities and even depression. They also damage the dopamine[1] pathways in the brain which can cause low and high dopamine levels in the brain. Low dopamine is responsible for the inability to focus, learning disabilities, and loss of coordination among many other neurological dysfunctions. High dopamine can cause hyperactivity, ADD/HD, obsessive and compulsive conditions and is also linked to schizophrenia. In children, usually first the high dopamine symptoms will appear as pesticides over stimulate dopamine pathways due to raising Acetylcholine. When the dopamine receptors "burn out" and down regulate as a result of over simulation children and adults can begin to exhibit the symptoms of low dopamine due to receptor down regulation and damage to this pathway. Discontinuance of conventional foods that are produced with the use of pesticides will reduce the demand for these foods thus the growing practices that produce them! There are vast wastelands in the farming areas of our nation due to

---

[1] **Dopamine:** chemical found in the brain and elsewhere in the body that functions asa neurotransmitter.

these very neurotoxic and carcinogenic products that kill all life it comes in contact with from the crickets to the birds.

Use all organic lotions for the skin and face. All conventional skin care products contain many chemicals that are both neurotoxic and carcinogenic. Transdermal (through the skin) exposure to these toxins are extremely potent in a damaging way to all organs of the body including the brain because they go directly into the blood stream gaining first pass exposure to all organs of the body before being neutralized by the liver. A very inexpensive method of nurturing the skin is using organic coconut oil with your favorite cold pressed oil / scent. The production of these toxins, the bottles they come in, and the toxins themselves bleed into our biosphere through many different avenues from the factory to the landfills they end up in.

Remove dairy and meat for two months to clear out old toxic saturated fats and provide a cleaner environment for detoxification. Conventional meats have a plethora of antibiotics, stimulant drugs, pharmaceuticals, and hormones in them of which many are neurotoxic. After that, consume only organic, pasture raised meats. The conventional animal for food industry is the most inhumane and one of the most toxic practices on earth today. Stop eating their products and put an end to animal suffering! If you are a carnivore, choose your meats from conscious organic farms that feed the animal what the animal was designed by nature to eat. Bugs and grass for chickens and grass for cows. Grains cause numerous diseases that the animal must suffer with including neurodegenerative conditions such as arthritis. And that is very painful especially when you consider the unnatural weight gain produced by the feed and use of growth hormones that they suffer. Also consider reducing your meat intake- you don't need that much. There are plenty of other excellent protein sources to consider. Balance your choices when it comes to eating animals with reverence. Lack of reverence for nature and all forms of life is what got us into this toxic mess. Reverence for our planet and all the minds, bodies and souls that live on it is at the heart of the Green Mental Health Care movement.

Remove grains which have gluten in them and reduce your general grain consumption. Grains are "inefficient foods" which clog cells and induce inflammatory conditions. Clogging cells is not a good idea because it inhibits the detoxification process and that is not good in this unfortunately toxic world. Grain production for animal feed (whom are not intended to eat grain) and humans supports a labor intensive, resource depleting agricultural model that drains resources that could be better focused in other areas such as organic vegetable, nut / seed, legume and fruit farming.

Discontinue eating Genetically Modified Organisms (GMO). These are food products that have been genetically modified via gene splicing and chemical alteration to produce their own pesticides and pharmaceuticals among other Frankenstein like goals. These pesticides are known to be neurotoxic; ergo, cause adverse mental health symptoms. Biotechnology led by Monsanto has literally opened Pandora's Box and no-one knows what the end will look like but it certainly won't be a healthy one. The body does not recognize GMO products as food and they are linked to birth defects and it is not hard to understand why. DNA transmutation is a fact of life on the planet. You are what you eat. These food products are so protected by news agencies held hostage by the companies that keep their lights on that people are effectively being kept in the dark regarding the extent of the dangers they present. Get educated about what you are putting in your mouth, body and brain! You can start at www.seedsofdeception.com and www.safe-food.org. The repercussions of Monsanto's and other Biotechnology companies scientists playing God in the laboratory could quite possibly cost us our planet—or the one we know and need to survive on anyway. They are producing a new and heightened level of toxicity in food which are directly related to mental health issues. The FDA has claimed it was not aware of any information showing that GM crops were different "in any meaningful or uniform way," from non-GMO crops and therefore didn't require testing. But 44,000 internal FDA documents made public by a lawsuit show that this was a complete lie. The overwhelming consensus among the FDA's own scientists was that GM foods were quite different and could lead to unpredictable and hard-to-detect allergens, toxins, new diseases and nutritional problems. It turns out that FDA scientists, who had urged superiors to require long-term studies, were ignored.

See: http://www.seedsofdeception.com/GMFree/GMODangers/FAQs/index.cfm. The production and use of GMO products is such an extreme act of terrorism upon human life and every single other life form including our planet that the positive impact on all living creatures through the discontinuance of the use of these products should be quite evident. In fact, stopping their production may be the single most important thing we must do to save the planet as we know it.

You must look at the ingredients of each and every box, bag, wrapper or can containing foods that you are considering eating. Look them up at the Environmental Worker's Group website www.ewg.org and be sure they are not toxic in any way. There are very few foods in packages or containers that are non-toxic. The best thing to do is to eliminate the middle-man and eat directly from the earth; whole, organic foods. There are over 40 different names for monosodium glutamate (msg) now. Again, you should eliminate all processed foods from your diet. Food manufacturers and distributors have license NOT to put over 1,500 chemical and food additives they use on the label because they are considered GRAS (Generally Recognized As Safe) by the FDA. The FDA also allowed Vioxx which killed 60,000 people into the consumer market and Aspartame which has a larger death toll and more complaints from anxiety and aneurisms to diabetes, seizures, heart palpitations and cancer than any other product ever approved for human consumption by the FDA. It has earned the crown in neurological symptoms complaints. A good place to begin your education on this chemical killer is http://www.321recipes.com/aspartame.html

The accumulative effects of these thousands of food toxins is devastating on every aspect of the life of the planet and the animals that inhabit it. I would have to write a mile long tome to explain the breadth and depth of the damage food chemicals have inflicted on our planet. These chemicals destroy life in and on the soil, water and wildlife in the air.

If you have a long commute to work, you can create a lot more Green time in your life by moving closer to work. This also eliminates the stress of the commute. This Green Mental Health practice reduces emissions and helps reduce CO2 emissions.

Purchase Green, non-toxic products for the home from environmentally conscious companies. This provides protection for you and your family from symptoms caused by the chemical assaults that are endured by the many, many neuro / excito and carcinogenic toxins found in carpets, paints, toys, plastics, and the thousands of other useless products people buy. It also redistributes the wealth in the country toward companies that are helping the planet away from people that are harming the planet.

Purchase only organic, non-toxic cleaners for the home and workplace. Also, encourage your local schools to do the same. The neurotoxins associated with conventional cleaners are linked to many mental health symptoms and even to causing asthma attacks. Please visit the Environmental Worker's Group for more information and this particular link regarding our schools:

http://www.ewg.org/schoolcleaningsupplies/overview.

Reducing the demand for these chemicals helps to reduce the chemical exposure and waste the planet is suffering from.

Replace aluminum pans with stainless steel or titanium. Preventing your loved ones from developing diseases such as Alzheimer's and Parkinson's which is associated with aluminum deposits in the brain, ensures a happier home which creates happier communities.

There is thimerosal in vaccines and flu shots. Thimerosal is mercury. Heavy metal poisoning is a direct contributor to adverse mental health conditions such as anxiety, schizophrenia, paranoia, panic attacks, addictive biochemistry and yeast infections which cause a plethora of mental health problems from chronic depression and anxiety to digestive disorders and cancer. It is strongly advisable to be tested for heavy metal toxicity and then if tests are positive, find a health practitioner skilled at chelation therapy. Chelation therapy removes heavy metals from the system. There are transdermal, oral and intravenous methods with varying treatment options within each modality. It is best to find and work with a knowledgeable health care provider to be sure it is done correctly and the metals are removed. Post treatment testing should be used to confirm success. Heavy metal contamination from our industrial waste, amalgam dental fillings, vaccines and flu shots, fish, and manufactured products is a major contributor to the death of ocean and all other forms of life. Also, if you live in a industrial area where there are many factories you absolutely must get a full toxic element test run to test for all toxic metals.

Do your best to eliminate the use of Styrofoam, aluminum and plastics. There are numerous toxins that bleed into your food from these products which contributes to the toxic overload in the body that is causing the mental health epidemic of today. Reducing the demand for these products saves the earth's resources and reduces the toxic overflow into our water, soil and air.

Of course this only serves as the tip of the iceberg in exposing the true impact in how your Green Mental Health strategy will save the planet, but it should be enough to make the simple point; that through saving your mental health you are saving the planet and all other living beings!

Now that you have taken the bad stuff out, here's what you put in: The pillars of excellent health

Organic whole foods: you absolutely must stay away from conventional meats from animals raised on antibiotics, hormones, stimulants, pesticide drenched feed, etc. These products were no good for the animal and are just as bad for you. The farms that raise these animals are corporations that have absolutely no value for their lives or yours. Animals are tortured by what the food, drugs, and conditions do to them and your health will be compromised as a result. Meat from sick and tortured animals can only make you sick and tortured by the symptoms their meat creates.

Clean, filtered water
Sunshine
Adequate sleep
Exercise – due to the unfortunate toxic overload poisoning our biosphere and us along with it, it is absolutely necessary to detox every day. It is advisable to exercise six days a week and on your off day take a sauna.

Basic Nutritional Therapy

- An organic whole food based vitamin
-
- An organic whole food based mineral supplement
- 3 to 5 grams of Vitamin C daily
- 400 mg. of CoQ10[22]
- Cod Liver Oil

Some Fundamental Treatments

Alkalizing your body. Yeast, cancer and colds prefer acidic systems and most people today are acidic. Many mental health symptoms are caused or aggravated by acidic pH.

Chelation Therapy: removing heavy metals from the body. Toxic levels of mercury, lead, aluminum and other metals are linked to many mental health issues today and many other toxic elements are developing into mental health issues as they accumulate in the body from various agricultural and___ industrial practices rear their ugly heads in our mental health. Amalgam (silver) fillings and vaccinations are the two most potent contributors of heavy metal toxicity and the symptoms that go along with them. It is also wise to consider getting the amalgam fillings removed and replaced with zirconium. I advise zirconium because composites have a mixture of less, but still toxic metals in them. Do not engage in professional (IV / suppository / transdermal) heavy metal chelation until you have all your amalgams removed! If you have amalgams and have chelation therapy you will leach the mercury from your fillings into your brain and body.

Infrared Sauna. Has clinically demonstrated to improve mood, kill bacteria, parasites, yeast and fungus; move water through the cells better by breaking water down into smaller molecular clusters and reduce inflammation. This is an excellent way to quickly flush toxins from the system that could be causing or aggravating your mental health decline.

More recreation and socialization—less TV and internet! Excessive television and internet use promotes sedentary23 and isolated lives. Very unhealthy for your mind and your body.

All of the above addresses the physical body that directly affects your mental health. However, you must also remove toxic people, relationships, situations, and work environments which also have a negative impact on your physical body which adversely affects bio/neurochemistry; ergo, your mental health.
Stress causes oxidative stress which harms all your critical organs and weakens the immune system. If you are experiencing any kind of chronic stress you must identify its origin and then create a plan to migrate out of it. If you feel you require counseling or guidance an excellent place to start is reading the first two free chapters of "Integral Life Practice" offered at http://www.integral-life-practice.com. It is what we use at my clinic in addition to Neurolinguistic Programming and these two very scientifically and evidenced based counseling / coaching systems have provided the best measurable results I have witnessed in helping people practice those lifestyle systems that promote

mental well being and create quality lives.

---

[22] **CoQ10 (Coenzyme Q10):** an enzyme produced by the human body that is necessary for the basic functioning of cells. CoQ10 levels are reported to decrease with age and to be low in patients with some chronic diseases such as heart conditions, muscular dystrophies, Parkinson's disease, cancer, and diabetes.

[23] **Sedentary:** a lifestyle characterized by a lack of activity or exercise.

Chapter 8
What to Do If You Are on Prescribed or Pushed Drugs

First, begin practicing the instructions found in the "What to Do If You Are Symptomatic and Not on Prescribed or Pushed Drugs" section and begin then to interview practitioners to find the Right Practitioner!

Important! You absolutely must work with a licensed and fully educated (in the areas I discuss below) health care practitioner to safely get off psychiatric drugs. They are toxic poisons that have skewed every normal, healthy biochemical process in your body and attempting to get off of them without caring, clinical supervision can present potential physical, psychological, and emotional harm to you and / or anyone around you. You also want to find a health practitioner that is accomplished in neuroendocrine disorders as this is the home of both the damage that led you to drugs as well as the damage that the drugs have done which stand between you and complete recovery; Green Mental Health.

One very criminal exchange between those on psychiatric drugs and their addiction enabling "doctors" is when they have tried to get off of them without the expert care of someone that actually knows how the body and mind works and knows how to help them do it correctly, as they begin to suffer the horrific symptoms of withdrawal and share their experiences with their "doctor" in hopes for help, the "doctor" will tell them that the symptoms they are suffering are proof that they are "sick" and need the drug. Nothing can be further from the truth! This is like telling someone detoxing from heroin or cocaine that their withdrawal symptoms are proof that they need the drug! Any time you detox from a drug you are going to experience withdrawal symptoms if you are not doing it with the support of a knowledgeable practitioner. You are not sick in the mind. Withdrawal symptoms are a product of the phase in- between the drug leaving the cells thus reducing the synthetic pharmacological effects they had on the body and mind and the body and mind responding with its own natural drugs in the form of neurotransmitters and hormones. This is why it is supremely important to supply the cells (body and mind) with all the raw precursors and the right environment for the body and mind to make its own natural drugs so that you may quickly experience the natural high- the product of Green Mental Health Care!

Definitions and Qualifications You are Seeking in a Practitioner to Assist you with Getting off of psychiatric drugs:

Choosing your practitioner may be the single most important decision in your recovery. A group of terminally ill patients who went into recession when all others had passed away were asked why they thought they had won over a disease that typically kills its host. The most common answer was "my relationship with my doctor".

Functional Medicine

(as described at www.FunctionalMedicine.org).

Functional medicine is personalized medicine that deals with primary prevention and underlying causes instead of symptoms for serious chronic disease. It is a science- based field of health care that is grounded in the following principles:
Biochemical individuality describes the importance of individual variations in metabolic function that derive from genetic and environmental differences among individuals.

Patient-centered medicine emphasizes "patient care" rather than "disease care," following Sir William Osler's admonition that "It is more important to know what patient has the disease than to know what disease the patient has."

Dynamic balance of internal and external factors.

Web-like interconnections of physiological factors – an abundance of research now supports the view that the human body functions as an orchestrated network of interconnected systems, rather than individual systems functioning autonomously24 and without effect on each other. For example, we now know that immunological dysfunctions can promote cardiovascular disease, that dietary imbalances can cause hormonal disturbances, and that environmental exposures can precipitate neurologic syndromes such as Parkinson's disease. (all of which can create mental health disorders).

Health as a positive vitality – not merely the absence of disease. Promotion of organ reserve as the means to enhance health span. Orthomolecular25 Medicine See http://www.orthomolecular.org

As conceptualized by double Nobel Prize Winner (Chemistry and Peace), Linus Pauling (scientist), "aims to restore the optimum ecological environment for the body's cells by correcting imbalances or deficiencies on the molecular level.

---

[24] **Autonomously:** existing and functioning as an independentorganism.

[25] **Orthomolecular:** of, relating to, or being a theory holding that mental diseases or abnormalities result from various deficiencies and can be cured by restoring the body's proper biochemicals, using such things as vitamins and minerals, in the body.on individual biochemistry, using natural substances such as vitamins, minerals, amino acids, enzymes, hormones and essential fatty acids."

Anything that influences the cell and promotes healthy cellular function is Orthomolecular Medicine. You must start with the biology of the individual. correcting biochemistry makes the "soil rich" for mind / body / energy therapies. Acupuncture, EFT, HeartMath, NLP, Cranial Sacral Massage, Chiropractic, skillful and gifted healthy lifestyle and practice coaching (such as that offered by the Integral Institute's

Integral Life Practice), counseling, etc. are all very helpful adjuvant26 therapies that engage and assist the healing process, however, if the body is poisoned and the biochemistry can not sustain healthy cellular functions you will not be able to receive the therapy well and it will not be able to initiate and sustain redirecting the flow of bioenergetics27 in order to align the cell to the subliminal28 laws of health and that is harmony with its environment. Basically you cannot be fighting your body and mind and experience any sustainable success with the very credible Green adjuvant therapies available. It is very difficult to penetrate an inflamed, clogged cell to correct its internal functions and it is also impossible to bring a cell to life that has no food in its environment to draw from to operate its internal machinery. You must also bring the cell into "growth" mode and that is the state of functionality that is able to use its nutritional stores for repair and replication rather than metabolizing toxins and mediating excess stimuli which puts an enormous energetic and nutritional tax on the body so thorough detoxification and replenishment of essential nutrition is fundamental to any healing event. Bringing a cell to growth mode also involves a stress-free environment as the cell cannot be in growth and protection mode at the same time. Just as your body's energy focus (where it applies its energetic and nutritive stores) is pulled away from digestion and nurturing the body when you are running from a tiger, the cell does the exact same thing on the microcosmic level. With no digestion, there can be no repair and replication, and without repair and replication there can be no healing.

All things that influence the cell in a way that assists its inherent wisdom to thrive; that is repair and replicate, is Orthomolecular Medicine, right down to how good that hug feels from your kid. Because there are so many "vehicles" of delivery (treatments) in Orthomolecular Medicine, diagnostics is extremely important. Your practitioner must be very skilled and knowledgeable in how the neuroendocrine functions in order to expedite the process of discovering what is wrong and then be able to successfully create a Green Mental Health strategy to treat the biochemical pathway/s that are deficient or "broken".

So Orthomolecular Medicine is Functional Medicine, however, you should be working with someone that is adept at exploring and exposing the root cause of your symptoms in the neuroendocrine system. Your practitioner should also know how the elements of nature (nutrition) will affect your condition and which ones are the most appropriate, ergo, the most effective for correcting the cellular dysfunction that is creating the bio / neurochemical dysfunctions producing your symptoms. Experience in Nutritional Neurochemistry is ideal as that is the science of how nutrition—both deficiencies and application of it is expressed in mental health. Targeted Nutritional Therapy is a science. It is not achieved by someone sitting across the table from you taking down your symptoms and then prescribing supplements. That is no more accurate than a psychiatrist doing the same just with toxic drugs. The only difference is, is that nutritional supplements won't harm, cause disease or kill you but you are still wasting your money by not hitting your target intention: Green Mental Health! Targeted Nutritional Therapy can only be achieved through rigorous laboratory testing and thorough exploration of your environmental influences- your lifestyle. You also want a practitioner that can orchestrate a targeted protocol utilizing the best of mind / body / energy healing techniques for your condition. One very important aspect of mind / body / energy healing is that since it involves the more subliminal energies of your being-ness it will certainly involve your belief system so that should absolutely be considered in selecting the right adjuvant therapies for you. If you believe swinging a sock full of dog dung will help you, you should be given the opportunity to swing dog dung over your head as many times a day as you feel is necessary. If it doesn't work, you will move on without feeling like you are being cheated of something you believe will help you. If it does help, great, let me know so I can add it to my repertoire of suggestions with my patients! I'm sure the comedy of the moment will be an adjuvant therapy in itself!

You want your practitioner educated, skilled, and gifted in environment toxicities and their impact on cellular function (such as toxicologists Doris Rapp, M.D. I also suggest reading her book Our Toxic World), biochemistry, neurochemistry, and molecular biology29. You want your practitioner to have a track record of proficiency in successfully getting people off of drugs and achieving Green Mental Health. What is also extremely important is that this practitioner not only listens to you but respects you and your body! Ideally, you want to work with a practitioner that is passionate about their work.

Remember, you want their qualifications in bio and neurochemistry to be focused on the functionality of the neuroendocrine system since that is what you are going to be fixing- your pharmacist within. Your internal pharmacy relies on your general biochemistry to deliver the raw materials your brain (remember, your brain is a full body entity with its crown on the top of your shoulders) needs to produce the neurochemicals in the appropriate quantities that make you feel good. And all of this is dependent on the cells of your body having the right amounts of amino acids, minerals, vitamins, and essential fatty acids to work with and the right "energy (chemically and energetically (stress) toxic free) in their environment to assist and manage the processes of health and well being. When your cells are able to repair and replicate they are happy; they are in harmonic resonance with their environment and because their needs for survival are being fulfilled you feel at peace and happy

---

26 **Adjuvant:** something that helps or reinforces a process, as in enhancing an immune response.

27 **Bioenergetics:** the study of energy transformation in livingsystems.

28 **Subliminal:** existing or operating below the threshold of consciousness but often being intense

29 **Molecular biology:** the branch of biology (study of life) that deals with the formation, structure, and function of essential to life at a molecular level, such as proteins, DNA, etc., especially with their role in cell replication and the transmission of geneticinformation. There is an innate wisdom built into your cells that is focused on survival- this

is why wounds heal without your intervention—thank God—we wouldn't know the first thing to do if we had to heal our own wounds mindfully- and remember that the next time you go to your doctor's office. How much do we really know about the human body and mind? Not much- so it is best to stick with, assist and respect the relationship it has developed with its environment over three million years to survive. Our utter ignorance is highlighted in conventional medicine's notion that it can control it with drugs. This notion is a big contributor to iatrogenic illness (death by medical treatment or procedures—including drugs) being the number one cause of death in the United States.

Essentially, you want Jane or Tarzan of the microcosmic bio/neurochemical jungle working for you; someone that knows how to navigate the fascinating world of those 60 trillion cells that are there simply to help you express the authentic you and enjoy the macrocosmic world you live in.30

Neurochemical

(from Wikipedia)

A neurochemical is an organic molecule, such as serotonin, dopamine, or nerve growth factor, which participates in neural activity. The science of neurochemistry studies the functions of neurochemicals.

Neurochemicals are found throughout the body as they pertain to nerve cells. The bulk of neurochemicals are found in the brain which presents the perception that neurochemical deficiencies are "mental" conditions when in fact they are products of deficient functions of the body and the brain and are most of the time created by toxicity, stress (over stimulated environment), and malnutrition. Do not be fooled by a full stomach. If you are not getting the nutrition your body and brain needs, you will suffer symptoms of malnutrition psychosis of which include many of the popular DSM "conditions." (The DSM is psychiatry's bible of get rich quick schemes they call the Diagnostic Statistical Manual).

———

Rehabilitation

To restore to an ideal functional state which is always the one determined by nature.

[30] Gary Null, Death by Medicine.

Orthomolecular Neurochemical Rehabilitation

The application of Functional Medicine (nutrition, mind/body/energy healing, detoxification, and environmental factors) to restore the health of the brain and neuroendocrine functions through clinically assisted detoxification, Targeted Nutritional Therapy (TNT), and creating an environment for the cells to heal and thrive which naturally corrects bio / neurochemistry.

All things that influence cellular development and function must be considered in a fully comprehensive treatment program based on the individual's personal biochemistry, environment, and lifestyle.

Stopping the toxic, destructive damage being done to the body and mind and providing a nutritive, non-toxic environment (this includes people, things and places), restores healthy bio and neurochemical functions, which by default, heals mental symptoms.

Remember, it is not all in your head! Better than 98% of the time there is an underlying physical cause to your mental health issues. The other 2% is reserved for actual birth defects, brain cancer, brain and brain tumors. There are now over 100 million people on psych drugs of which 98 million do not need to be. In fact, neither do those that actually have the actual brain health issues stated because it has been established that even those people would of course have better therapeutic outcomes using non-toxic, non-invasive and non-addictive; Green therapies as opposed to toxic psychiatric drugs!

First Goal: Detoxification and Stabilization with Minimal Withdrawal (transitional discomfort)

First, find a Functional Medicine Practitioner that is formally trained in Orthomolecular Neurochemical Rehabilitation (ONR). ONR is what practitioners like Dr. Abram Hoffer, M.D., Ph.D., Dr. Joan Mathews-Larson and myself practice. The science of ONR brings together scientific DIAGANOSTICS to define the appropriate clinically assisted detoxification, organic whole food diet, dense nutrition using vegetable juicing and first chain foods (chlorella, chlorophyll, blue/green algae), Targeted Nutritional Therapy (TNT), very helpful adjuvant services such as Neurolinguistic Programming, Integral Life Practice / Recovery coaching, Acupuncture, colonics, Infra Red Sauna, Lymph Drainage Massage, Chelation Therapy, Cranial Sacral Massage, EFT, Cranial Electrical Stimulation, and the practice of Environmental Hygiene through identifying and eliminating all sources of neuro and other toxic influence in the person's food, drink, personal hygiene, home, work environment etc. All things that influence your cellular function must be explored and corrected in order to achieve true healing and sustainable mental health. The more you eliminate oxidative stress (free radical damage) to the brain and other critical organs charged with the care of your mental health, the better and faster you will heal.

To pull all internal and external environmental influences together on all levels of your psychological, emotional and physical being-ness and align them with your personal goals of health, career, personal fulfillment and beyond, I personally and professionally employ the Integral Life Practice model. For my patients, the coaching begins with a focus on readapting to life experienced by the authentic you. When the fog of legal and illegal addiction lifts it is a brand new world and most people need guidance in how to migrate through that world with their own vision, wants and needs at the steering wheel. We then apply the health, insights and inspirations you develop as you heal into a Integrated Practice of excellent lifestyle skills that are there only to function as enablers of your highest vision that you create for yourself. For further review of this extremely effective coaching therapy that brings all areas of your life together and in alignment with what you want out of life, please visit Ken Wilber's www.integrallife.com.

ONR requires a deep understanding of Functional Nutrition, neurochemistry and the neuroendocrine system. It is the network of endocrine glands and how they are able or not able to respond to the messages of the nervous system and the functional chemistry of the brain (primarily influenced by the external environment and the feedback system of the neuroendocrine system) that is the home of the root cause of all ill mental health symptoms except for genetic abnormalities which represent less than 1% of mental health issues. A genetic link would be one which demonstrates that DNA damage exists and that has even been proven to be helped if not corrected with ONR treatment. Even those mental health symptoms that arise from DNA abnormalities will express themselves through the neuroendocrine system that provides a roadmap right to the root of the problem. The science that has established that the environment of the cell is far more predictive of the cell's health or dis-ease than the gene is called "epigenetics." Epigenetics has proven that your genes do not control the destiny of your health. So that means there is a Green Mental Health Care solution for 99% of you and hope for increased quality of life and possible resolution of symptoms through Green Mental Health Care for the other 1%.

Remember, this is a life or death decision many times because if you choose the wrong practitioner, and that would be one that is minimally qualified or one that practices nutrition but has little understanding of how to create an environment for the cells to thrive or nutrition applied to neurochemistry and the neuroendocrine system, you won't achieve the sustainable mental health you seek and more dangerous, you may lose hope.

By the time you are done reading this book, you will know all the right questions to ask. If the practitioner you are interviewing cannot answer them with confidence and the answers do not resonate with you and what you have learned to be true, move on. Also, if they try and move you into another direction, that means they are not qualified in this field but still want your business so they will try and talk you into their treatments based on their limited understanding of Functional Medicine applied to Orthomolecular Neurochemical Rehabilitation.

The laws that dictate health are not negotiable. Just as you cannot grow roses in a toxic waste dump, you cannot expect to derive personal enrichment, growth from life's experiences nor quality of life if you are poisoned. Psychiatric drug toxicity literally disables your ability to respond in a healthy way to your environment, cutting you off from the natural flow toward good known as 'grace'. This is where your mental, physical, and situational suffering begins: opportunities for a healthy and productive life are lost because your vision is blinded by the inner chaos caused by drug toxicity.

To get well, you must detoxify and provide a nutrient rich, toxin free environment for your cells to repair themselves and replicate which will correct the biochemical chaos that is creating your symptoms.

Green Mental Health Care, the Medicine of the Future that Saves the Future!

Green mental health care is non-toxic, non-addictive and non-invasive care of your mental health and it has proven to provide superior outcomes at a fraction of the cost!

It is our intention to provide a safe and informative solution oriented place to land where true compassion, respect and care for each other translates into each and every person who is not on drugs but symptomatic finding the path to true freedom from the mental health symptoms that are epidemic today and if they are on psych drugs, detoxing, and repairing the damage, discovering excellent sustainable mental health and reclaiming their authentic self and lives from psychiatric drugs.

It is the responsibility of our government to use tax payer money to offer and provide those services in the public health sector that do not pose health risks and possible death and instead provide solutions known to increase quality of life and success rates. In today's public mental health care system true Green Mental Health Care strategies such as dietary education, toxicology education which would help you identify what is truly driving people crazy these days such as aspartame, MSG, pesticides etc., exercise programs, acupuncture, good functional counseling instead of compliance coaches, colonics, yoga, tai chi, and detoxification programs are not offered. To date, it is supposed to be illegal to force drug a person. Well, if they don't offer any alternative to toxic psych drugs for today's epidemic mental health issues, isn't that a form of forced drugging? Our public mental health care system is actually against the law!

Green Mental Health Care; How to Get Off & Stay Off Psychiatric Drugs

It is imperative that we refocus mental health strategies away from mind-numbing, disease and death causing methodologies as the pharmaceutical companies are acquiring so much power in our government that US citizens are now being force drugged- including our children. As soon as the people began educating themselves and turning away from psych drugs, the drug companies targeted children- especially foster children, pregnant women, and the elderly in convalescent homes whom they feel society is least concerned about. These populations are now facing forced and coerced drugging meaning that human rights such as education and other medical services are being denied if they do not comply. Other people that want to get off are being threatened by their doctors with hospital admission- psychiatric incarceration. Parents are losing their children to foster homes and being charged for medical neglect and child endangerment for refusing to give their children psychiatric drugs that have been linked to child suicide, cancer, diabetes, sudden death, obesity and violence.

Pharma – Psychiatric agenda, we must demand that these services be offered and exhausted before drugs can be considered.

Remember, medical practice and philosophy is supposed to be rooted in a "First, Do No Harm" consciousness! Bring the Care back in Mental Health Care—say no to Big Pharma profits and medical regulations and yes to Green Mental Health Care for all citizens!
The human consciousness is the collective consciousness of the biosphere. We are fully integrated with all living beings and our planet. If our planet is suffering, so will we and that suffering will be reported by our consciousness or what we call our mental health. We must practice Green Mental Health in order to save our minds, our bodies and our planet. It's time to shine—for ourselves, for each other, for the planet.

In service we shine,
Shine!
Genita M. Mason Lic: H.H.P., N.C., M.H. Medical Director, The Biosanctuary

Orthomolecular Neurochemical Rehabilitation Website:
www.thebiosanctuary.com
Email: FindPeace@biosanctuary.com United States
877.285.92

RECOMMENDED READING

These are must read books that go into great detail regarding the damage environmental and food toxins do to our cellular functions from the energy producer, the mitochondria to our DNA and the mental and physical health that suffers as a result.

Our Chemical Lives And The Hijacking Of Our DNA [Dec. 09], author Catherine J Frompovich delves into the effects of a chemical-laden world on the body at a cellular level.

Our Toxic World: A Wake Up Call author Dr. Doris Rapp, M.D. Toxicologist.

There is also an excellent report titled Multiple Chemical Sensitivity: Toxicological Questions and Mechanisms which goes into great detail as to how neurotoxic chemicals create neurological disorders.

Theo Colborn is the Senior Scientist with the World Wildlife Fund; she is an expert in endocrine-disruptive chemicals; co-author (with Dianne Dumanoski, and John Peterson Myers) of Our Stolen Future–How We Are Threatening Our Fertility, Intelligence and Survival–a Scientific Detective Story. This book explains that since the early 1920's, mankind and industry has released thousands of chemicals— over 500 of them have been found at harmful levels of concentration in human tissue
—which were never there before. Many of these chemicals, some of which are passed from mother to child in the womb, can interfere with the "chemical messengers" which "tell" the body how to develop, and eventually affect the human nervous system, endocrine system or immune system, potentially affecting the health, development, behavior and intelligence of any human, anywhere. You can listen to her interview with Amy Goodman at this link:
http://www.democracynow.org/1996/3/15/toxic_chemical s_that_threaten_us

———

Mike Adams, on NewsTarget.com provides this report on over 100 toxic foods chemicals, most of which are neurotoxic:
http://www.naturalnews.com/026244_food_MSG_neurotoxins.html

For further information visit the Environmental Worker's Group at www.ewg.org and the Environmental Health & Toxicology from the National Library of Medicine at http://sis.nlm.nih.gov/enviro.html